Mending *the* Broken Heart

Mending the Broken Heart

A JOURNAL TO WHOLENESS

Joan Conkey

To order additional copies of this book, contact:
Xlibris Corporation
1-888-795-4274
www.Xlibris.com
Orders@Xlibris.com
116274

Contents

MENDING THE BROKEN HEART

A Journal to Wholeness

—DEDICATION—

This book is dedicated to my husband, Howard, and my great-grandson, Greg, two guys who showed me how to have fun and put so much joy in my life!

Acknowledgement

My deepest gratitude goes out to all who have shared their grief, their joy, and their recovery with me. Knowing each of you has made a difference in my life.

Preface

It all began at a summer institute for alcohol and drug abuse counselors in Austin, Texas in 1983. The University of Texas was the home for that annual institute for many years and my husband, Howard and I, were introduced to a learned and intuitive person who would later teach us a process that would be a part of the healing of so many broken lives. We had been into our own personal recovery from alcoholism and codependency issues for several years and were, at that time, working in the field professionally. When we first met him, he told us that he had heard of our work in the *Valley and he was interested in expanding his work, which he had started in Houston, Texas, and expanded to other locations. We also were aware of the work he and a colleague had been doing.

My first response to this suggestion was a pleasure at being included in this plan and feelings of inadequacy. Although we had both worked in the field of chemical dependency for some time, we had no experience in the formalized process of setting up an out-patient treatment program. Our mentor immediately soothed our fears by letting us know that the staff he had in Houston would take over the major part of all that. He wanted us to become trained in the process of this type of therapy, hire, train and supervise other counselors, and operate the program in Brownsville. It had been operational in Houston for a couple of years and had been quite successful.

Indeed, he had hired some exceptional people in Houston to do the therapy work, using this process, and it seemed to be a great opportunity. Indeed it was. We turned that corner of our lives not realizing how much impact it would eventually have on us and so many others.

*The Rio Grande Valley in Texas extending from Brownsville to Mission—along the border of Mexico.

In the following pages, I will try to explain how we started using grief resolution therapy in Texas, how the group process works, and various means of increasing the effectiveness of the process. The last part of the book will include personal stories of people who felt the quality of their lives enhanced by the use of this type of work. In less than two years, it became clear to us that we needed to change our fields of professional interests from commercial real estate and education to our newly discovered interest in the recovery from chemical dependency and its impact upon family members. I joined the ranks of academia once more, moved forward into certification, licensing, a graduate degree in education with specialization in guidance and counseling. There were so many early leaders in the field that had a great impact on me. The early work of Wegscheider, Satir, the Johnson Institute, Kubler-Ross, Jacqueline Small, and Rev. Joseph Kellerman, contributed tremendously to my understanding and skill of working with people.

During my thirty years of working in the field of substance abuse, I have worked in several capacities: as a director of a council on alcoholism and drug abuse, as the clinical director of an out-patient program addressing the needs of the chemically dependent and families, and as a co-founder and developer of a school based student assistance program which identified, referred, and gave support to students who were substance abusers or who were living in homes in which the use of chemicals or abuse issues had created problems in their lives. For several years I have used journalizing, and grief groups, and found them to be highly effective in combating the devastation left behind in the path of the addictive process.

The original family intervention process which was developed by the Johnson Institute is significantly important in terms of how it teaches family members to address their feelings, confront the denial in living with chemical dependency, and to communicate long—suppressed feelings of sadness, fear, confusion, and anger. Joining with others for support and finding a safe place to do this work is extremely important. The chaos brought about in families who go through these changes is often extremely difficult and often permanent without ongoing support.

All I hope to accomplish is to describe, as best I can, what the process is, how it works, and what I have personally found to be effective. I believe I have taken knowledge and the process and put my personal fingerprint upon it. After reading this, I hope you will do the same. None of us does it exactly alike. This book is only a basic recipe; you add your own special ingredients to make it be just right for you.

"When the shell of
my heart breaks
open, tears shall
pour forth and they
shall be called the
pearls of god."
—Rumi, 13th century poet

MENDING THE BROKEN HEART

A Journal to Wholeness

Brownsville, Texas, a city of approximately 150,000 inhabitants became our permanent home after spending the first forty years of our lives in Northeastern Kansas. My husband, Howard, and I moved there in 1976 after beginning our own recoveries from alcoholism in the previous year. We had absolutely no idea of what was in store for us as a result of the changes brought about through recovery and moving to the southernmost tip of Texas. What a joy the last thirty years have been! The Menninger clinic in Topeka, Kansas, helped us begin our journey. Our six weeks of treatment there introduced us to the world of therapy, twelve step programs, unlimited relaxation techniques, the huge relationship between mind, body, and spirit, and opened the door to a wonderful healing process. We have had the tremendous opportunity to pass along some of this healing to others.

Many were there before us and many will come after, but my deep gratitude and thanks are daily in my mind for having my husband, my partner, friend, and lover be a part of this journey with me. We had the experience of sharing our disease for twenty years and then we had thirty years of sharing recovery. We consider ourselves extremely fortunate in this respect and do not receive this gift lightly.

Whatever we have been so freely given, we wish to pass on to others who come after us.

I have nothing new to tell you in this book. Emotional, physical, and spiritual healing has been addressed by many for thousands of years. I have nothing original to write about. If you have read or studied anything about this subject, you know how many people have written books, made tapes, given lectures, purported to be THE answer. I do not claim to have THE answer. What I do believe is that there is a therapeutic process that I will refer to as *grief resolution therapy*, and that will be a combination of various theories and techniques that I have found to be extremely valuable and practical in dealing with grief and loss as it relates to addiction and family members of addicts.

We received extensive training in Houston, listening to lectures concerning chemical dependency and its impact upon the family, sitting in groups with therapists using the process, reading, listening, and absorbing all we could. The process itself seemed so easy, so natural—as it still is. Learning how to apply it and fine tune it continues to be a challenge and a joy! For the first time, I began to understand the grief process was a part of living in a dysfunctional family. I began to truly understand the enabling process and why family members continue to do that, in spite of themselves. I began to be clear about the disease and I began to see true healing from the disease in some new ways. Using personal and existing theories and models, formed a process that was not to be completely recognized to the full extent of its importance for many years to come. We worked with some very skilled clinicians in Houston and learned a great deal.

We soon opened an out-patient center in Brownsville and began using grief resolution therapy as a method of helping chemically dependent people and their families resolve grief and heal. This grief process dealt with the trauma that had occurred in a person's life and that it did not matter whether the trauma was a result of a spouse's alcohol consumption last Saturday night, or whether it dealt with the trauma of an adult child of an alcoholic who had been sexually abused by her father thirty years before. The process worked to heal the wounds.

Placing the words that express what happened in written form and then sharing that pain verbally in a small safe group of people is what this process is really about. The only magic is in that process itself.

The liberation and expression of the feelings of what happened allow the individual to release the pain and move on. So what makes this process so different? Terry Kellogg* says that we must have "safe harbors" in which to come to grieve, must connect deeply to others, as well as be able to see how that trauma impacted us and how we continue to act it out in our lives today. The process allows for the reality of the trauma to be addressed but does not end there. This process allows the client to identify losses from the traumatic event, grieve those losses, as well as identify one's own coping mechanisms and acknowledge those as being either damaging or healthy. Then the process of addressing change in those behaviors can be made.

— What happened?
— What did I lose?
— What did I do to cope?
— What did I lose or gain as a result of that method of coping?

Done properly, this process allows a client, in his own time and space, to work through any painful event and release the energy from that pain. It might be viewed as an in-depth fourth and fifth step, following the guidelines of Alcoholics Anonymous. The group provides a "safe harbor" and the therapist becomes a navigator who guides and acknowledges. Every navigator or guide has his own special touch to add but the purpose of this writing is to put into words, as clearly as possible, the map to follow. Within the parameters of this type of therapy, clients are able to develop abilities to support, nurture, and claim themselves again.

The miracles I have seen come out of these groups are truly astounding and I feel so very privileged to have been a part of this process. It has added a dimension to my own life that I never would have believed possible but for which I am very grateful. My purpose for writing this book is to allow others to learn and continue to use this process that was given to me.

*Terry Kellogg, Broken Toys. Broken Dreams.

*Alcoholics Anonymous—Steps 4 & 5

Being a part of others' change and growth has helped me beyond my ability to explain or express. While writing about this process, I lovingly release the outcome of how and where it will be used. I write this by pen and the written word, not by computer or word processor, because I want the added element of feeling and the reality of feeling for myself as I write it. That gets distorted as it is processed through machinery, so I'm doing as I tell my clients. "A word of caution to those who will use this process: never underestimate the power that this type of therapy carries. It is very powerful, and the use of it has a very strong effect on clients. My hope is that the process will be used with a great deal of personal responsibility and respect for the power that it carries.

Therapy is defined by Webster as *remedial treatment of bodily, mental or social disorders or maladjustment.* As we know, therapy today comes in so many forms. The process of one human being helping another along a path of self-discovery or healing can be done with a mere smile, which takes only a second, or by psychoanalytic process, which takes years. I have a belief that there is no one specific way of delivering effective therapy. I believe it depends upon the specific needs of the client and to what extent that client may be open at any given time. We, as therapists, must be open to learning techniques that will fit the individual at that particular time in his life. I will not go into a discussion of all the different therapeutic approaches or make comparisons. I will make an effort to describe this process and how it works.

GRIEF RESOLUTION THERAPY is basically a three phase process. The first portion is the "telling of the tale" in which the client, outside of group, writes a series of incidents, in letter form, addressed to the person who has been involved in the pain of an incident. For example, a client may have had a painful series of incidents with a spouse. The client would be asked to write a letter somewhat as follows:

Dear Dave,

Last Christmas when your parents were here visiting, you promised to meet us for dinner at Gios at 6:30. You never called and you never showed up until later at home that night. I felt angry, anxious, unimportant, responsible for your parents, resentful, and worried.*

The incident is read to the other group members and they in turn have the opportunity to give feedback as to how they might be feeling if it were to happen to them. This serves as a validation and a support for the feelings of the reader. Many times that client's feelings were unacknowledged at the time of the event, either by self or others.

One at a time the client reads a series of these incidents. How many can be read at a time depends totally on the depth of pain of the incident and how it impacts the client and other group members. No matter who is actually reading, all group members are "working" and are involved in the process. A group can only deal with so much pain at any one time and the therapist must be in touch with just how much work can be done in one session. Sometimes a client will read several incidents all at once or sometimes only one incident will be read, depending on its impact. For example, if a client reads an incident which elicits a lot of shock or anger, it will be necessary to process all of those feelings by whatever means necessary. The specifics of feeling facilitation will be addressed later.

After all incidents have been processed, which normally takes several weeks, the next step of the group process is to place these incidents on the first portion of the matrix. (See attached—Illustration #1).

Since the group has already heard the incident in its entirety, it is necessary to place only a brief summary of the incident in the first column. The second column includes all of the feelings that were written when the incident was shared in the group. The third column is to help the client state and claim her value system that was contradicted by the incident originally. The group can be a very valuable asset in finding and stating what appropriate behavior would have been at that time rather than what actually happened.

Clients are requested to have a loose leaf notebook and to write each incident on a separate page. They need not be written in chronological order at the time of the writing but will be placed in chronological order before they are put on the matrix. The matrix will be more fully explained later.

Examples of appropriate behavior of incident #1 might be:

— My husband is considerate
— My husband is punctual
— My husband values my feelings
— My husband is responsible

The fourth column deals with the losses that were experienced by the client as a result of the contradiction. In this case there were several losses such as:

— trust
— role model of a husband
— fun
— family togetherness
— self worth

The group, at this point, helps the client identify and grieve through these losses. The recognition that these losses had nothing to do with the client or behaviors of the client is important to validate at this point. This is an important part of the work as it is here that the client begins separating her identity from the identity of the "abuser" and no longer continues to carry the responsibility or the guilt in response to the incident. The fusing that had taken place between client and the "abuser" is at this stage breaking up. Realizing that the client is in no way responsible for the actions of the abuser is an extremely important and freeing part of the work.

Illustration 1

The Incident (WHAT HAPPENED TO ME)	My feelings about it	The way the behavior contradicts my value system	Losses resulting from this contradiction	My reaction to the incident and behavior	The way my behavior contradicts my value system	Resulting losses to my personal identity

*She and her are used as pronouns here only because the greater percentage of my clients have been women. The process is the same for men.

Each stage of journalizing work is to be fully completed before moving on to the next stage. For example: The client needs to write and read *all* incidents on a specific relationship before putting them in chronological order on the matrix. These will be read and worked all the way through before the client moves on to the second portion of the matrix work.

On the second matrix the client begins to identify her own actual behavioral responses to the trauma of the incident. It is in this column that the client looks at sometimes irrational or self destructive behaviors that may later result in becoming repetitive compulsive behaviors. They are frequently found to be enabling behaviors such as covering up, lying about the incident, minimizing what happened.

They frequently become "numbing" responses such as over-working, gambling or over-eating, use of chemicals, beginning an affair, all of whose purpose is to shut down feelings. These behaviors may be immediate or they may be somewhat delayed responses. Each client will need to identify these responses *without* self judgment. At this stage of the work, there is a shift from focus on the abuser to focus on self. It is of *utmost* importance for the client to hear that these were behaviors that were the best she could do at the time. Some may have been in contradiction to her own value system, and if this is the case, those are to be recorded on the second column of matrix #2. (How my behavior is in contradiction to my own value system).

Examples would be:

— I am honest
— I confront appropriately
— I share my feelings appropriately
— I am alcohol and drug free
— I am faithful

The last column is for identification of the losses as a result of one's own behaviors. Some examples of these losses are largely, but not totally, internal losses such as:

— self-trust
— self-esteem
— health
— hope
— dreams

They can also be relationship or systemic losses such as:

— healthy communication
— fidelity in the marriage
— role model of a wife or mother.

The corresponding layers of grief are later explained in more detail regarding the process described above.

The length of time that it takes to complete this process depends upon several factors such as the size of the group, how quickly trust is built between group members, how long the client was exposed to the abusing behavior, how severe the abuse was, how much ongoing abuse is still occurring, and present day coping skills. Many factors contribute significantly to the length of time it will take to work through the trauma. The development of defense mechanisms were essential to the survival of the client, but also need to be gently confronted in the group process.

In my groups, I have used grief resolution therapy with both men and women. I see no reason why the process would not work for adolescents if they are truly motivated to do the therapeutic work, but I believe there is a certain degree of maturity that is necessary for this to be a productive course of healing. I have done groups with only men, only women, mixed, and one very homogeneous group of Mexican American women of age 30-40. This is by no means a valid cross-section of what might work, but, I will tell you what has worked best for me.

I did a men-only group for several months and it was working, but what started out to be a group of five soon dwindled to three and I decided to add women. The men who stayed in the group appeared to be able to emote better with females in general. I cannot say that this was a specific gender issue. It may have been trust issues that just took time to develop, but the group, in general, did better as a mixed group. On the other hand, all women groups do exceptionally well. Deep levels of trust develop in those groups and catharsis is frequently the norm for women in these groups. I have no way of knowing if facilitation by a man would make any great difference in a men's group or not—perhaps so. Or perhaps this only upholds what I have understood for years to be true and that is that men do better, in general, in mixed groups, while women do better separately.

The relationship between client and the person on whom the client is writing varies greatly. I have had clients deal with the painful behavior of husbands, wives, ex-spouses, parents, their own children, siblings, aunts, uncles, grandparents, friends, lovers, employers, and institutions. It doesn't seem to matter a great deal what the relationship is; the process works equally well for all. The only criteria is the client's willingness to be honest and the level of willingness to grieve and let go of the pain.

There have been some clients that had difficulty with the process. These are people who continue to use chemicals from time to time. Perhaps they may not have had enough sobriety before they began the process (if they were chemically dependent to start with). Normally, I would recommend at least a year of sobriety before a client begins family of origin work. This will give some time of stabilization in the client's program of recovery and help him focus on the immediate goal of staying clean and sober. I have worked with some recovering individuals sooner than a year, but for the most part, I believe it is a good idea to wait until the client is stable and secure in sobriety.

The best group size, I have found, is from five to seven people. Good work can certainly be done with as few as three but I have found that if I have six or seven in the group, there will likely be at least two people out on any given group day due to illness, vacation, business, or being out of town.

The length of time of the group is one and one half hours. It is important to begin on time and end on time. It does happen from time to time that catharsis is going on at the time group is to end. I try to handle that by helping the client pull back together as soon as possible after closing time. Occasionally, I have asked the group members if they are willing to spend a little more time after closure with the group to ensure the emotional safety of the client who has been heavily into a grief process.

Normally, I open the group with a request that members share whatever feelings have been predominant for that week without getting into a long explanation of the week's events. There is a tendency for clients to want to focus more on the present than to get into the past pain so it is necessary to frequently remind group members that we are to focus primarily on the resolution of past issues. With most of my clients, I find there are many on-going and present issues that can occupy the time and emotional energy of the client if not deflected. I remind clients that the present issues need to be addressed either in individual session, with a sponsor or friend, and it is recommended that they go to a twelve step group for ongoing support. I find that regular participation in twelve step meetings is an extremely important part of the recovery process. The healing of the client is smoother and quicker with the use of twelve step groups on the outside.

How long the healing process takes depends upon so many factors that is difficult to say how long a client will be working in the group. It could take months or years depending upon such factors as:

— how long each separate painful relationship existed.
— the urgency with which the client moves into the work
— the depth of the pain of the incidents and for how long the abuse continued.
— the level of trust in the group.

Time to read and process in the group is usually shared equally with the group members themselves deciding whose turn it is to read on any given day. It is very infrequently that a client takes more than his fair share of group time. On the contrary, it is more often that group members will urge one another to "read today" or confront a member who appears to be "falling behind" in her reading. Normally two or three persons will read at each session. It is important to know and to remind the group members, however, that everyone is working in every group even if they are not reading. Each member becomes involved in the feeling levels of the reader, generally with a great deal of empathy and personal responsiveness. This is an important element for the therapist to understand and to facilitate effectively.

This is done by personally being able to be spontaneous and in touch with the emotional levels of the reader and reacting appropriately. A therapist also helps by requesting expression of feelings by the listening group members, frequently and regularly.

Example: The group member of the above incident may have read what happened in a monotone voice with very little affect although when asked she may have reported feeling angry. It is then important for the reader to receive the feedback that she is incongruent. What she says she feels is not matching with what she looks like she's feeling. Group members can be helped to point out that "Sally says she feels angry but her voice is low; her eyes are wide. She appears to perhaps be feeling some shock and disbelief even though she says she's angry."

As mentioned before, trust between the members of the group is extremely important. Support of each group member at all times is primary to the success of the process. Ensuring safety of the expression of feelings is absolutely essential. No feeling is ever wrong.

A word about memory: the resounding pain of it on a regular basis, or the lack of it, will be an issue in the groups. It has been my experience that it matters very little exactly how much the client remembers. As the process evolves, he/she will remember exactly what, and how much they need to remember to heal. The sharing of group members' experiences will quite frequently trigger memories in other group members' minds. Actually it is a good idea for all members to keep a pad and pencil handy to make notes when a memory is triggered. This is a very important part of the process and very valuable in the business of retrieving repressed memories. I treat any memory as being valid for the client and the expression of those feelings attached to it as valid.

Occasionally, a client will be reluctant to do this type of group work, fearful that he/she will not be able to remember enough to heal. Such a case was "Juanita", (names are changed to protect confidentiality) but when the time was right for her, she was able to remember all that was necessary for her healing. There are other clients who have such a flood of painful memories that they are afraid of being overwhelmed with the pain of recall. It is important to assure these clients that they will be able to work through all of those memories in a timely fashion. In these cases, I have found it very important to help the client really stay focused and centered on living in the moment. Pointing out how strong she has been to survive all of that for years is important. I try to help them do the work they need to do in group and then find a way to safely put the rest on a shelf until the time comes to do more. They need to know that they do not have to do all of this work immediately. It took time to get to where they sought help and their healing will come in the appropriate time also.

Now a word about how clients go about the process of sabotaging their own treatment. Within each of us is a desire to heal and move on in a positive way with our lives but at times the fear of change far exceeds the desire to change. When this fear reached a certain level, a client may, without even realizing it, begin to sabotage their own treatment. There are several ways they may bring this about. Some of the following are frequently heard statements of reasons to discontinue the process.

I can't afford it.

I have too much work right now.

I have too much pressure right now.

My therapy is interfering with my program.

My sponsor says I need to focus on today.

All of that is in the past.

I need to move on with my life.

I need to take more night classes and there is a schedule conflict.

I am not living with him/her anymore so I do not need to work on this anymore.

These are only some of the reasons heard for discontinuing therapy. These all seem reasonable and valid to the client. I certainly honor their right to continue or discontinue their process, but I do ask them to look at the real reason they are choosing to discontinue. I ask them to look at the progress already made and encourage them to examine their fear about continuing. Many times it is because the client is getting close to dealing with a difficult issue and will use all sorts of avoidance techniques rather than face the issue, without realizing what is happening. Many times the client will find the courage to move on past the fear if safety and a non-judgmental attitude can be taken by the therapist. Sometimes the client may need to discontinue the process at that time because it is not right in terms of timing. I do frequently remind the clients in groups that it takes a lot of courage for them to continue to discover themselves and I acknowledge them for what they are doing for themselves.

What happens in terms of mental and emotional process with clients in journalizing groups? The grief stages will be acted out, sometimes several times at different levels.

For example: A client may come in with a lot of anger, then find themselves going into shock as they realize the substantial number of losses they have incurred. They may move again into anger, either toward the perpetrator of the abuse, toward herself, God, the disease, or everything in general. Knowing that the anger is important and not to be overlooked is a part of the healing process. It has been said, jokingly, that clients need to wear T-shirts that display a warning like, "Caution! I am in a journalizing group, subject to change at any moment!"

There will be moments of denial, disbelief and numbing. These are natural parts of the healing, to be honored, never trampled upon. Eventually the client will come to a place of true acceptance of what has happened to them and a healing with the past that will allow them to move on in their life, make better choices, and honor themselves and their feelings in a new way.

I do not believe that a client has to completely forgive a perpetrator or forget what happened. I do believe that it is important for them to get a different perspective on what happened, expose it, feel the feelings, and come to realize that they did the best they could at the time (as did the perpetrator). The working through of the grief helps them to move out of a victim role and move on to be more in charge of their life from that point on.

During the actual process of group each week, different modalities may need to be used to facilitate feeling levels. I believe in using whatever works as long as it does not harm the client or others in the group. I keep several "tools" on hand at all times when I do a group, such as pillows, a blanket, large towel, sponge covered bat, small plastic bats (child's baseball bat available at most toy stores @$1.89), large stuffed animals, different sized chairs, including a small but sturdy plastic child's chair. I also have in my office an old, good sized hassock (foot) stool, padded with foam, and covered in a tough naugahyde material. We almost threw it away several times because it is not an especially attractive piece of furniture, but it has been invaluable as a receptor of clients' anger. From multiple blows from bats, to fist pounding, to screaming words of profanity, it has stood up over the years as a wonderful and irreplaceable piece of therapeutic equipment.

In my therapeutic approach I use whatever seems to fit at the moment to facilitate a client through the feelings. I use Gestalt technique a great deal. Role play and reversals are important. Playing out the power issues via "tug-of-war" with a towel is very helpful when the client can realize all she/he has to do is step out of the power play rather than continue to engage. I also use guided imagery as a tool, but with caution, always giving the client choices.

We may use imagery at the same time, always supplying lots of positive support if she goes into a past painful experience. Asking her to take along powerful, positive and supportive friends to protect her is an important step in this work. I would strongly recommend the therapist have a good foundation in imagery and safe hypnosis technique if it is used at all. This is not a normal part of this group work but it can be used to enhance the process if it is done carefully and safely.

I have found that trust levels are better established if some of the following are adhered to:

1.) The group meets at the same time and in the same place. The only time we do not have groups is Thanksgiving, Christmas, New Year's time. I try to arrange my vacation time so that groups do not have to miss more than one week. To still have my own needed time off, I take more frequent but shorter vacations. This is always established well in advance.

2.) When a group member needs to miss a session, she is asked to inform the group as much as possible in advance. If an emergency arises, she is to call ahead of time and let the group know.

3.) Group members are sometimes asked to pay a month in advance for the group. This tends to encourage regular attendance. If reasons are valid for missing a session, such as illness, the client is given credit for a missed session for the month.

4.) Group members are encouraged to exchange phone numbers and be in touch with one another. The normal restrictions concerning no dating among group members applies but I have found that the mutual support in between group sessions can be quite valuable.

5.) An *extensive* description of group and its expectations is done before the client ever enters group. I want the client to understand the process and be aware of the commitment that will be necessary. Group work is not for everyone.

6.) If a client has proven to be disruptive in group for any reason, this is dealt with through open communication. I have infrequently found it necessary to remove a client from a group but there have been times when that was needed for one reason or another. Changing a client to another group is infrequently necessary but has also happened.

Most of the clients I have worked with do not know, or have never learned ways to support other people or what to expect in terms of support. This is one of the benefits of this type of work. The modeling is actually done by the facilitator. It is then copied by the clients. It involves such things as active listening, accurate feedback, showing care and genuine concern for others, appropriateness with voice and touch and consistency. As these are demonstrated over and over again, clients are then encouraged to put these to work in the process of the group. After these skills are learned, the process of facilitation becomes much easier and the process proceeds much more smoothly. What skills are learned in group are then put to use by the client outside the group with family, friends, and co-workers. Communication skill development is a big and important by-product of the group process. Since most of these clients come from families that did not know how to communicate or support non judgmentally, to confront lovingly, and to express feelings openly, these lessons are critical to establishing a better quality of life.

Does this process work for most people with different types of relationship problems? Yes, I have seen it happen that way. I have worked with a twenty year old in the same group with a sixty year old, and all ages in between. Interestingly enough, the issues with all dysfunctional relationships seem to be so similar in nature that it makes little difference if it is a parent, child, spouse, relative, or friend. Within the group there is always someone who can relate or learn from the position presented. As a matter of fact, some of the most insightful experiences have come from group members who get to take a look at "what it was like for that other person" in the painful relationship. I mention again, that it is very important for the client to have sufficiently recovered from any personal substance abuse issues before moving into this therapeutic work. I have seen it work to the detriment of the client if he or she is still carrying a lot of guilt as a result of the addictive disease and tries to do relationship issue work before he or she is adequately recovered.

I would like to say a word about homogenous groups in terms of other than gender issues. I facilitated a group of young Mexican American women, all between the ages of thirty to forty, in varying states of separation or divorce from abusive husbands. The group formed an immediate bond and a good level of trust. As a result of that, several began to become friends outside of the group and socialize on a very regular basis. It was not long before a "clique" developed in the group and some dissension developed. The group then needed to spend some of group time sorting through all of that instead of moving ahead with work. In the long run my belief is that it would be better to not have a group with so much commonality even though, at the time, it appeared to be of great value. It appeared to me that it slowed down some of the process of the group.

I later had another group, that, although they were diverse in age, became very close. They had dinner together upon occasion, called one another between sessions, and were tremendously supportive of one another. They actually moved forward rather quickly as a result of the bonding that occurred between sessions. It is important for the facilitator to have a good feel for the group, be in touch with and sensitive to what is happening within the group.

Frequently a childhood role, such as mascot or hero, will be played out in group. The time will come when the facilitator will be conscious of this and help the client also to be aware of the role and to make decisions about continuing or not continuing with that role.

Seeing how they continue to live out childhood roles in their adult lives is frequently helpful in determining change.

Taking responsibility for personal change is a big part of growth in a journalizing group. It is not a matter of blaming one's parents or spouse for what happened. It is about realizing that there were no other choices for the client up to a point. Once the awareness is there, then begins the process of developing enough support and implementing the coping skills to bring about the necessary changes for a more successful life.

I have seen in my practice that sexual abuse victims will consistently push away from healing and come back again. It is almost as if they are challenging the therapist to test whether or not the therapist will be there for them on an ongoing basis. Trust issues become pressing and recurrent when dealing with groups of this type. For this reason, the on-going need to model consistency and support is ever present for the facilitator to demonstrate. Self-care is essential.

A therapist must not take on anyone he/she cannot, for whatever reason, be comfortable working with, or stretch themselves past a point of comfort, time-wise or emotionally. Being in touch with one's own limits and capabilities is essential in this work. If the therapist finds himself/herself dealing with issues in group that he/she has not personally resolved, it will quickly become clear and the therapist must address these issues within himself. Failure to do so will injure or slow down the process of the group.

The ways the therapist can meet their own needs are exactly the same as what the client needs to be doing. We must "talk the talk and walk the walk". The following is a list that I have found helpful and have needed to refer to on an on-going basis:

— Time off pursuing outside interests.
— Twelve step support group meetings.
— Exercise
— Personal Therapy (individual, marriage, and family when needed).
— Massage Therapy.
— Prayer and meditation.
— Supervision, that is, getting regular feedback and support from another professional so that healthy perspective can be maintained.
— Stress relief by means of talking, writing, self-hypnosis, etc.
— Participation in workshops, seminars, and growth enhancing experiences
— Practice self-affirmations.

I don't believe in asking a client to do anything that I have not done or would not be willing to do myself. It frequently takes a lot to maintain one's own health and emotional balance while doing this work.

A very important discovery that group members make while doing this work is about value systems. They will discover that, over the years, their own basic values have been compromised again and again. As a result of growing up in a dysfunctional family they may not have had values established, such as a right to privacy, a right to be heard, a right to their feelings, or a right to be supported and nurtured.

When dealing with adults, it is frequently helpful to get in touch with these values by making reference to what they want for their own children. It is often easier to be in touch with what my child deserves or has a right to expect than what I desire or have a right to want.

This helps the client see the personal damage done, grieve that loss, learn to find ways to be personally responsible for meeting one's own needs and/or connecting with safe and trustworthy people that will help meet those needs. It is, at this point of awareness, frequently helpful to do some inner child work, helping the client see himself/herself as a child in need of support and love.

Acknowledging this child and its needs, teaching the client how to meet these individual needs, is a large part of the healing process.

Valuable ways to bring this about include bringing a picture of self as a 2-4 year old child to group, guided imagery that will help client see self as a perfect little boy or girl, or role play that allows adult parts and child parts of the client to interact in healthy ways.

Establishment of an emotional connection between the spontaneous and feeling parts of self and the wise, mature, and objective part of self will add a balance and will direct the person to a sense of wholeness. Building upon positive aspects of the self, affirmation of growth and change, and the complete acceptance of the client's feelings, as they are, makes possible unlimited growth experience.

To make groups a safe environment for all clients it is imperative to work with them individually long enough to be assured that they are going to be capable of functioning in the group appropriately. Those with severe mental illnesses, on heavy levels of medication, or who may not be able to control their rage will not be appropriate for this type of group experience. Careful screening will help safeguard the group and avoid the problems associated with having to withdraw a client from group because the client is unworkable.

As a client progresses through the layers of grief he will become aware of and experience three types of losses. They are personal loss, interpersonal loss, and systemic loss. On a personal level such things as joy, safety, money, dignity, and time might be lost. On another level of interpersonal or relationships, losses might be boundaries, companionship, healthy sexuality, or role model of a spouse. On another level, involving the entire system there is a third level of loss experienced. This is defined as systemic loss and include losses such as family pride, family unity or family dignity.

Frequently, if the client is still in a relationship with the person on whom they are writing, they will begin to make different choices about their own behavior in that relationship. As they grow in their capacity to self-nurture they will find they have gains rather than losses as a result of their own behavior. This supports the philosophy that we cannot change anyone except ourselves. Once this happens, the client finds it increasingly difficult to stay in toxic relationships and endure the losses associated with those relationships.

Upon completion of the last matrix it is frequently helpful to make a list of his/her own behaviors that seem repetitive and compulsive.

Once this is done, the client may deem it necessary to step up support for changing some of these. For instance, if the client found he/she used excessive work as a coping mechanism, a plan to set up a healthier schedule and follow that with a monitoring process would likely be helpful. These discoveries and the associated commitments to change are the pay-offs for this work.

One other very helpful component of this process is to ask the client to write a letter of good-bye to the person with whom he/she has had a painful relationship. This is an emotional good-bye letter, not always a physical good-bye. This frequently puts additional closure on the process for the client and appears to be a means to further release the client from any lingering enmeshment. Some samples of good-bye letters are included in the following section.

At some point in time the client has discovered, worked through, and resolved the grief surrounding the relationship. At this point, the client sets some new personal goals which include a commitment to self care and self-nurturing. As the individual experiences himself as worthy and deserving, he is capable of self acceptance and self love.

He has learned he is deserving of attention, love, honesty and healthy relationships. As the client continues to support those new belief systems, they do indeed become an integral part of his life experience.

To those of you who will move forward into this grief resolution process as a facilitator or as a client, I wish you well. You are truly courageous people stepping into a difficult and challenging process.

There will be hours of great pain, but always accompanied by growth.

Go well with peace and love.

The following are some personal stories of individuals who have gone through this process. They describe why they joined a grief resolution group, how it worked for them, and the changes brought about as a result of that experience. These people share their experiences in an effort to deepen an understanding of the process and to provide hope for those who are still struggling with unresolved grief.

"There is sacredness in tears. They are not the mark of weakness, but of power. They speak more eloquently than ten thousand tongues. They are messengers of overwhelming grief . . . and unspeakable LOVE."
—Washington Irving

—Marlene, Janet And Jackie—

THREE GENERATIONS

I've had an opportunity to work with many people, many families, but one that brings back many memories is of the three generations of women that crossed my path. Marlene was in her late fifties when I met her. She'd suffered from chronic alcoholism for years, struggling with frequent relapse. I was not able to work with her in group but I did some individual work and she made efforts, time and again, to stay sober. She was from an Irish family, had twinkling eyes, and a bright smile when she was sober. When she relapsed into her disease, she turned into a different person. She was surly, angry, and distant. She had one daughter, Janet, that she loved very much but they struggled in this relationship. There were the lies, the promises broken, and much hurt. Marlene died of her disease at age 66, but her daughter, Janet, as the result of working on her mom in group, was able to let go of much of the pain she'd experienced for years growing up. Janet had a daughter, Jackie, and I began working with her as a teenager. She desperately wanted to break out of the familial patterns. Her mother had achieved continuous sobriety for many years and Jackie began the difficult task of sorting through her emotions and the devastation of her family's history. After a couple of years in a journaling group, she began to heal. She'd never known her father but she believed it was important to learn about him and how his absence had affected her life. After locating him half way across the country, tracked by computer, he invited her to come and meet him and his present family. She continued to be in touch and learned more about her heritage. This young woman was spared from alcoholism in that she didn't drink. She did, however, find herself attracted to men who were abusers and emotionally unavailable. She finally pulled out of that level of her life, returned to college, working for the local newspaper. She was a talented writer who is still moving forward to improve her life. Lives are never perfect in recovery but she does have tools to deal with what she faced as a child, losing her grandmother to the illness, struggling to grow up with a single mom, and coming to grips with her own future.

All of these three women were very bright, witty, and a delight to know. It was a great blessing to be able to know them and walk the road of life with all of the three. Jackie now has a little girl herself, now 2 years old who can already express her feelings verbally and appropriately. She is adored and loved as life goes on.

—*Juanita*—

Juanita came into treatment at age 39, never having been married, the oldest of six children, and the daughter of an alcoholic. She reported that all of her siblings have work addiction except for a brother who is alcoholic. Upon entering group, Juanita struggled with a severe lack of memory. She finally, managed to get down a few incidents from her childhood. Being the oldest in her family, she carried with it a great deal of responsibility for the family during the drinking years and even more after her father died, Juanita was eleven years old. The initial writing carried with it a lot of embarrassment and shame for father's behavior when drinking. It was much later in recovery when she began remembering bits and pieces of her father sexually abusing her. The experience of attending a workshop for abused children triggered some of her own memories approximately four years after she had begun therapy.

Dreams had always seemed very real to her and her memory was triggered also by a regular pattern of dreams involving entrapment and fear. Juanita had a great deal of fear about sex and had been very limited in her life concerning sex with men. In her mid forties, she began having some memory of her aunt and then her father having sexually abused her. The memories came in small bits. She described them as a succession of photographs. Often the smell of alcohol or the roughness of her father's beard were triggers for more memory. Later the memory of an uncle raping her also came. At this point Juanita slipped into depression and needed temporary inpatient care to deal with her issues. Still more memories of another uncle's abuse of her were to be discovered. After her month of intensive care, she returned to her home, emptied of much of the rage she'd carried for years, armed with additional tools of recovery. Since that time she has resumed a full and useful life as a teacher and later married. Juanita gives most of the credit for her recovery to the safety of her therapy group. She used the group process off and on for approximately five years. Ten years after her initial entry into recovery, she still attends twelve step meetings for on-going support.

She occasionally slips into old patterns of compulsive obsessive behaviors, but, for the most part, her live is full, happy, and productive.

—Becky—

I was brought up in an alcoholic home and I really believed my family was normal. I thought everything was perfect, but that was not reality. As the oldest of eight children, (four boys and four girls), I became the good, responsible, obedient daughter. My mother relied on my help as well as my sisters. However, because I was the oldest, my name was always called out first by my mother for doing anything she needed, and believe me, there was plenty to do. I hated coming home from school to mountains of dirty dishes to wash, piles of clean laundry to fold, and various other household chores. I had no time to relax or even do my homework. I was quiet and compliant, but underneath it all, I was building resentments. We were Catholic and I did everything I was told to do just like I had been taught at home and in religion classes. It was never expressed directly, but I think my parents wanted me to be a Catholic nun.

When I was thirteen, I remember crying about not wanting to be a nun. I felt God wanted this. My mother assured me I didn't have to be one, but I thought that was the only way to get to heaven. I was feeling so crazy and couldn't talk about my fears to anyone. I stuffed my feelings about this as I did all my feelings. Then, there were my parents' fights. I don't remember so many before I was six, but they began to happen more often as I grew older and especially during planting and harvesting seasons. They were physical and verbal fights. My dad would come home late from drinking and/or working and my mother would attack. You never knew who would get yanked out of bed to be attacked by dad. There was a lot of anger. I prayed that God would help but he never did. I was a scared, shy, nervous teenager who eventually ran off with a boy. My parents hated that I got married. I didn't see my family for more than 2 years. Although, my sister was going to college at the same campus, she avoided me. I was sad. With my husband's help and support, and his father's help, I received a teaching degree. I was so proud, but my parents were more interested in my sister's wedding which was happening at the same time as my graduation. I missed the graduation to be in my sister's wedding. However, I still wasn't good enough because they still didn't accept my husband. My husband completed college and we moved. I became pregnant and after I had the baby, my husband left me for another woman. I was devastated and weighed less than 100 pounds. I married and divorced two more times after that. This had all happened in my 20's. Deep inside, I knew something was terribly wrong with me. No one else in my family was divorced. Then when I was 29, my mother suddenly died after falling at home during another of my parents' drunken, alcoholic fights. On the gurney, as they wheeled her out of the house to the ambulance that horrible night, I smelled alcohol on my mother's breath. My mother who supposedly never drank. Died of two massive strokes ten days later. I was an emotional mess. I blamed my father for her death and everything else. I was in such shock and I hated him so much. I couldn't prove anything, but I knew dad had had something to do with her death.

In my thirties, I began my search for help. A friend of mine who knew my story suggested I go to Alanon. I didn't go. I went to therapist after therapist. I got involved with yet another man and was beginning to see a pattern. I began to realize there was something wrong with me. I had blamed all these ex-husbands, boyfriends, and family members for my messed up life. I finally attended an Al-anon meeting when I was about forty one. Little by little, I began to change. I stopped drinking alcohol and I found out about therapists who were also involved in 12-step programs. I was scared and ashamed, but I knew I needed more help on a one-to-one basis than the meetings were providing for me. I contacted some therapists, I'd been told about in my Al-anon group. I needed help and I felt calm talking to them. At last, I felt there was hope. I began working with a therapist who finally understood alcoholism and all its effects. After several individual sessions, I began group work. I felt comfortable in my first group which was made up of women. I worked the matrix (something like a fourth step inventory, but more thorough and intense). I dealt with my father, mother, and the three ex-husbands. It was painful and I had trouble with being on time and sometimes not going at all to group because I didn't want to feel the feelings. My therapist never gave up on me, even though, I didn't think I was worth becoming healthier and better. In group, when I read painful incidents that had happened, I wanted to leave and not see anyone in the group that heard the horrible things I had done or had allowed to be done to me. I didn't give up and I kept going and going back to group. Then, I had to change therapy groups and it was going to be a mixed group, no longer women only. I was feeling just crazy. I felt that most of my problems were caused by my involvement with males. I was sick about the change. I balked and balked at attending this new group. I hated it. There were a couple of women, but I couldn't stand the men. To top it off, one of them was a Catholic brother. I had had such issues with the nun thing.

But God works in mysterious ways. He knew who I needed in my group to help propel me to a higher level of recovery. Over time, I got better at accepting these men. I began to change and acquire a different prospective. Being in the same group as the Catholic brother helped me overcome my fears from childhood over being forced to be a nun. It was liberating and a miracle. I ended up liking the men as just people, not men who just wanted to sleep with me.

Yes, they had relationship issues, sex issues, emotional issues, just like me and I could relate to them and they could relate to me. I felt comfortable with these men and I never thought that could happen.

God helped me through all these wonderful people to forgive myself, forgive my family. I did the best I could at the time. However, because I stuck with my recovery all these years, I am a better, more confident person. I was in group therapy for a total fourteen years. I don't care about the time, because I believe that slow motion gets you there much faster. I'm still not completely well, but I probably never will be perfectly recovered from all the effects of alcoholism. I am a work in progress. The point is, that I am a much happier and healthier person. I wouldn't have done it any other way. I am so, so grateful to my therapist who truly is the main reason I stuck with this recovery process. She is truly one of the kindest, gentlest, but firm people I've had the privilege of having in my life. God put her and her husband in my life when I needed someone. I could have easily blown my head off, I was so down and depressed before meeting them. I am so much happier living my life now and am so very grateful to have found recovery.

—James—

My name is James and he is an addict.

Steven Covey operated on the 90/10 rule. 10% of life is made up of what happens to you, 90% of life is decided by how you react to the 10%. We have no control over the 100% of what happens to us, but we can control how we react.

I did not get into recovery voluntarily but rather waited until my life had become unmanageable. I was spiritually, physically, and emotionally bankrupt. I had covered multiple addictions until at forty eight years of age, my cover was blown. I was having an affair and could no longer control my drinking or lying to cover up. I spent sixty days in in-house treatment facilities and came away with enough understanding to know who my actions had hurt and who the true victims were. My addictions were selfish and isolating. Exactly opposite from what I really wanted: to be included and affirmed.

A few years into counseling, I was invited to join a group to begin journalizing. I listed what happened to me, what my reaction was, how that was different from my value system, and what my gains and losses were with each event. Journalizing allowed me to see how I had given my power over to people, places, and things. Parents, siblings, children, and my wife were all included in my list of people

I chose to work on. I learned by listing my gains and losses on paper, I had done a good job of minimizing my entire life. I was not allowing myself to have feelings or healthy boundaries. Through journalizing, I learned that I have the right and obligation to protect myself with healthy boundaries. I have also learned to identify my feelings and healthy ways to react to life's challenges. Journalizing helped me to make peace with my parents before they both passed away. All the anger and resentment finally made sense and I could deal with it as an adult. Before they passed, I was able to forgive them and accept them as they were.

With my children and siblings, I began the process of accepting them for who they are and working on not controlling them.

I am thankful my wife has gone through the same process. We understand each other better now. We have a healthier relationship now and we do not try to change each other.

I owe a great deal of the peace and understanding in my life today to my journalizing counselor, my beautiful wife, and the process of journalizing.

I will forever be grateful for the second chance I was given and for the members who shared with me in my journalizing group.

—Phyllis—

I have been sober since September 8, 2002, but I suffer from co-addiction and co-dependency. I am married to a sex addict.

Before seeking counseling for myself, my husband and I went to a counselor in a nearby town. He taught me about co-dependency and recommended I read <u>Codependent No More</u> by Melody Beatty. I read that book and found myself on many of the pages. I learned from these few counseling sessions to let go. I learned too well how to let go. I focused on my career and decided that I would become the best teacher and mother that I could be. I found a job I loved, and I had wonderful children so my life became about them . . . to the detriment of my marriage. My husband and I grew apart. I was oblivious to the distance because I was happy in my little world. I let go of trying to control his behavior. He found comfort in porn and flirting with other women. In 2002, I found a receipt for condoms that were purchased while I was in Europe on a two week trip with my son. We don't use condoms because my husband had a vasectomy. It was obvious that my husband had purchased them because there were other things on the receipt that he uses. At first he denied purchasing them. I struggled all day with this lie, and at 10 p.m., he finally admitted to the purchase. I insisted we attend counseling. We began seeing the author of this book.

During our first session, he admitted being a sex addict, and we began the unending dance of addict and co-addict. This was an extremely difficult time for me as my sister was dying of stage 4 breast cancer, and my mother was diagnosed with pre-Alzheimer's disease. I was learning all about sex addiction and was scared to death. I started taking anti-depressants, which helped my anxiety. We struggled through counseling for about four months, and my husband continued with his porn use. I insisted around the first of January 2003, that he check-in to treatment or the marriage was over. He left for the Meadows on January 3. On January 30, my sister passed away. We all attended the funeral and then left for family week the same day. My children were only able to stay for 2-3 days and then returned home. It was during family week that I learned my husband had an affair with his secretary. After returning home alone, I continued to work in counseling, but now my focus was to either become strong enough to live with an addict or become strong enough to leave. It was at this time, I started the group journalizing program. I needed validation that my husband's behavior was wrong. I needed to tell someone what I had gone through.

I joined a group of women who were married to sex addicts and/or were addicted to their relationship. They shared their experiences, their reactions to these experiences, and their feelings about these incidents. They also explained how the incidents contradicted their value system. These women shared behaviors that, in some cases, were similar to my behavior, and in other cases, were very different from my life. I had my eyes opened to lives that were much more abusive than mine, which was good for me and my victim thinking.

After a few weeks of listening and observing, I felt strong enough to begin my own journaling. Once I began writing and sharing, I found a support system that I never had in my life. I had never shared the ugly and emotionally abusive experiences I had endured with anyone because I did not want to endanger my husband's standing in the community or with my family. I protected his reputation like a good co-dependent. These women listened to me and supported me when I cried. They understood that I did the best that I could. After I shared all of my husband's behaviors, I could think that scarred me emotionally, I started over on the matrix and began looking at what I did during these experiences. I had to admit to some ugly behaviors that I exhibited to cope with my pain and embarrassment. This was the first time that I thoroughly examined my behavior and how I contributed to my co-dependency. It was truly eye-opening and extremely painful at times.

After I wrote about my husband, I then wrote about my mother, father, and sister. I learned how I became the woman I became. I saw the patterns of my behavior starting back when I was a small child. I was (and still am) amazed how I was programmed to marry the sort of man I married and to respond to the abuse I received. I spent about 4 years journalizing my way to an awareness of how I had become who I was. I also learned that I can change how I react to people and their emotional outbursts. I have also learned how to separate my crap from their crap.

I learned that I can change my behavior and thus change my experience. It is a daily struggle because learning a new way to live is like learning to write with my left hand after writing with my right hand my whole life. I have to live consciously and think about feelings, experiences, and words.

My husband went through the journaling experience too. I am sure that we would not be together had he not. We both learned about our families, our behaviors, and our ability to change. We still struggle, and I expect that we always will, but we respect each other on a level that we never had before.

—Barry—

I am an 84 year old male and I have been sober from alcohol for 29 years. My father was an alcoholic—his father was and so was his father. I hated alcohol. I never intended to follow in his footsteps.

My mother was a bible carrying Baptist and there was no alcohol allowed at home. When I was 3 years old, we moved from the city I was born in, and moved 1500 miles away. We lived in one room together for several years and after I started school, we moved about every time the rent came due. My father worked 17 hour days and we took his lunch and dinner to him. I say we, because I was an only child and there was no one to leave me with. When we would pick him up at night, he was usually drunk and they would start fighting over something or other. We finally got a trailer to live in behind the business he ran by himself. As I got older and he had a car, my mother would take me with her when he didn't come home and when we found him all she would do is tell me, "look at that, I hope you don't grow up like he is". My mother also told me that she was going to divorce him, but I came along and she had no way to support me.

At 13, I started drinking and the very first time I did, I got drunk. I drank off and on through high school. I then spent 2 years in the Air Force, 11 months overseas. I drank there as well and got drunk quite often. I came back from the service and 13 of my friends went to a college a long way from our hometown. When I registered for the first time, they asked me what I wanted to take and I said "something easy". I had no idea as to what I wanted to be. No one ever told me I was going to have to support myself. My other friends graduated and I was still there. I only went to class to take the tests. I had a number of female relationships and they always were beautiful women. I was only interested in looks on the outside. I realize now I had no clue as to who I was. I had a convertible car at school., fine clothes, and plenty of money. My mother made fun of that and were not well to do.

I lacked 9 hours to graduate when I quit school. I went home and started working for my dad in his hardware store. I lived at home and I kept drinking, not every day, but quite often. Of course, my dad and I didn't get along and I was unhappy but couldn't break away. This went on until I was 27 years old. I woke up one morning and first thing, looked outside to see if my car was there and it was. Then I looked in my closet and saw a number of tailored made suits. I had a diamond ring on my finger, my car was a Lincoln and also an electric start engine on my boat. I said, "I have all of this and I am miserable". I went back to church and my relationship with my father got much better.

In a few years, I got married and we had two children. After 8 years of marriage, I came home one night and my wife said, "I want a divorce. Our children were 2 and 5 at the time. She moved 550 miles away, but 30 days after the divorce, she tried to commit suicide. I had to go bring the children back to where I was living. After 2 years of therapy for us both, we married for the second time. Then she wanted a third child which I tried to talk her out of. She was on the pill and without my knowing she became pregnant. I was so angry but I said to myself, well it has happened so I stuffed the anger. From that time on my life went downhill. My back began to hurt more and more so I had to take darvon for it. As time went on, the pain got worse and I took more and more pills until I had a hard time doing anything. Then I studied some drug books and found that amphetamine drugs would give me energy, so I tried them and they did. I bought them from a drug stand in Mexico, they were cheap and plentiful. This went on for several years and I ran a business, but I am sure I was not much of a businessman or a father. I was always on the go, but I had trouble sleeping. So, after a while, I started drinking and taking pills. I got really bad and my wife flew me to Dallas and I was put in the same hospital that she had been 10 years before. I spent 3 months there and came back and didn't take pills. But, I did drink from time to time. As time went on, my wife said she wanted a divorce, which we did and the oldest 2 children came to live with me and the youngest stayed with her.

I would drink off and on and it got less often but the degree of it got worse until I was forced by the manager of my business to do something about it. She found this couple that she heard about and I agreed to go. It was something I wanted but also didn't want. They suggested I go to treatment but I wasn't about to do that again.

Finally, they suggested I go to A.A. meetings. I went and I heard something about God and I had been looking for him my whole life.

So, I went to 5-7 meetings a week, but I didn't feel any better. These same 2 people started me on guided written therapy. You chose your mother and father and others in your life to write on, one at a time. You write an incident in your life, starting as a child, which you can remember. Then how you felt about it, how it affected you and what your losses were due to this happening to you.

I wrote on my mother and father and both of my marriages to the same woman. This took a number of years for me and each week we had to say what feelings we had. This was a problem for me because I had no idea what I was feeling. I was afraid to be angry because I was afraid I would lose control. I couldn't cry because when I was 3 years old my dad told me "a dime for every day you don't cry". Doing this therapy was the most painful thing I have ever done in my life—but it was the best thing in my life. I saw that I was

abused, that I didn't feel safe in this world, that I had no
self worth or self-esteem and no identity. I did not know
who I was, what I wanted, or didn't want. I continue to go
to meetings and slowly but surely, I am beginning to love
myself for which I am grateful to journaling and the people
that have shared their lives. I have shared mine, my life
now is not perfect, but now I am not a bad person. That
I am an addict and will be the rest of my life and I must
take care of myself and rely on a power greater that myself
whom I chose to call *God*.

—*Yolanda*—

My name is Yolanda. I first sought counseling in my early 30's after experiencing my first panic attack which landed me in the emergency room at 2:30 in the morning. I thought I was having a heart attack. Once the hospital staff examined me and gave me the "good" news that it was not a heart attack but an anxiety attack, they suggested I see a doctor for a follow up. The doctor then recommended that I see a therapist to figure out what the cause of my anxiety might be. The first counselor I saw helped me figure out that there was some trouble in my marriage that might be causing the panic and anxiety that I was experiencing but it really didn't provide many answers for me. My anxiety grew and I started losing weight and feeling very shaky and vulnerable but I still had the worst ahead of me. About a year later, my marriage was over and my husband moved out leaving me with our 4 year old son. My father, who was my biggest ally was diagnosed with cancer and given no more than 6 months to live. If I had ever felt lonely before, it was nothing compared to this. I felt like my world was falling apart. My mother and I didn't have the best relationship. She and I had butted heads consistently since I was a pre-teen. I guess we were both fighting for queen status in our household. Being that she was the adult I guess she won out most of the time which made me angrier. I saw her as my competition for my father's attention. It always seemed as though it was my dad and I against my mom. Well now it was time for me to grow up. I could no longer run to my father for comfort because he was facing his own fears and struggles. It was at this time, that I decided to try counseling again. I was referred to the author of this book. I worked with her on a one to one basis for about 6 months before I was put into a new group that she was forming. I felt very fortunate that I had met 2 of the other 3 women in that group at a codependents anonymous meeting and had just bonded, so from the get go, it felt safe to be a part of this group.

The first person I worked on was my husband, since that was the relationship that had led me to therapy again. It helped me to realize that as sorry as I was feeling for myself because of the break-up, I had a lot to do with it. My husband and I had married because I was pregnant. Neither one of us was in love with the other but we thought we were doing the right thing. Shortly after we were married, we experienced a lot of problems. We were both immature and felt like we had been trapped into marriage by the other. About a month after we were married, I miscarried. At that time, I thought God was trying to tell me something and I wanted to end the marriage but was scared, so we continued with the facade, It lasted ten years, produced a son, and some good times. However, toward the end of the marriage, I had stopped functioning because of my anxiety and prayed that my husband would find another woman so that he could finally leave me alone. Well that wish came true, but instead of being happy, my ego took over and convinced me that he had done me wrong and I played the sympathy card for as long as I could. Fortunately, after doing the work in therapy, I was able to own up to my end of the demise of the marriage and I was able to let go of the self-pity. It took me a good year, year and a half, but I worked beyond the fear of raising my son on my own and became a better mother because of it.

The second person that I worked on was my father. I realized that my father was an active alcoholic most of my life. While several of his friends had stories of my father fighting after getting drunk, I never saw that side of him. At least, not physical fights. I did see and hear him get into verbal arguments with my uncles and some friends when I was young, it never escalated beyond that. Being his only child and spoiled rotten by him, I always took his side and felt sorry for him. I thought he was the greatest father and I felt that I had to protect him from my mother and any others who criticized him.

I took on the role of protector and he let me. My father was good at playing the victim. Maybe that's where I learned it from. When he got home after drinking, my mother would usually get upset with him and she would raise her voice to him. My father would play the victim and tell her that she was the reason he drank and that he would love to run away and live on his own where no one would give him a hard time about his drinking. Afterwards, he would tell me that if it wasn't for me, he would have left my mom a long time ago. I always felt that I was the glue that was keeping my family together and that if it wasn't for me, my dad would be gone and I'd be stuck with my mother. That gave me a sense of power that was never really there, but when you grow up hearing statements like that, you tend to believe them. In my case, I certainly did, and that made me walk on egg shells so that my father would never get upset with me and then actually leave us. It also gave me a reason to feel resentment and anger towards my mother. I thought that she was evil and that because of her I had to be twice as good to keep the family together.

Taking on that responsibility made me feel important and resentful at the same time. It provided me with a very false sense of reality.

While I was writing on my father, he passed away. It was very difficult to continue the work without feeling guilty that I was talking about my dad after he was gone. I felt that I was betraying him somehow. However, I knew that just like with my ex-husband I would feel relief when I finished and that it would give me a better perspective of what was real. That's just what it did. I realized that my dad was a beautiful person, but he had been emotionally stunted because of his drinking and that he had been unable to take responsibility for his actions. Therefore, it was easier for him to blame my mom and to allow me to be the referee than to accept that he had a drinking problem and own up to the problems in the family because of his drinking. I was able to forgive him for allowing me to be the middle man and for taking on a responsibility and a false sense of power that should have never been mine in the first place.

My mother was the third person that I wrote about. This relationship to me was the most difficult one to deal with and to write about. My mother had been a very over-protective mother but she was also the disciplinarian. As I mentioned before, I had a love/hate relationship with her. I hated that she was so over-protective and that she was the one that seemed to always say no. Plus, she was the one that spanked me and grounded me whenever I did something wrong.

Feeling that I was tough enough to protect my father and feeling that sense of empowerment, I didn't feel that she needed to be so overbearing. Our relationship always felt like a power struggle. I guess without knowing it, we were fighting for the queen bee role in the household. One, which as a child, I never should have had but felt I had earned. It wasn't until I got older and married and was out of the house that the relationship with my mother began to grow and become more mature. When I became a mother myself, I realized where my mother was coming from and why she might have done things the way she did. I still didn't agree with all of it, and still had bitter feelings towards her. However, because of the journalizing work that I did, I was able to be more accepting of it and of her. I also realized that while she might not be changing anytime soon, I could. Having the awareness that came about with the journalizing, I could react differently and make a shift in how we interacted. After all, my mom was now a widow and getting older and we were two single moms. She was the mother to an adult daughter and I was a mother to a young male child and I needed her in my life and I wanted for us to have a good relationship for the sake of my son. It took a while after finishing my journalizing to sort through the residue of feelings that I experienced and I was lucky that it brought a new and more positive attitude towards my mother. It has not been perfect, but I am so grateful that after all these years, we have a more loving and respectful relationship than ever before. Three years ago, she had open heart surgery and came to live with me. That was something that was pretty scary for both of us but thank goodness, when I put into practice what I have learned, it makes for a smoother ride. I don't know how things would look like today if I had not done the work on my mother that I did more than 15 years ago. Our day to day life, living together, would have been a hell on earth for both of us. Thank God that while we might have bad moments, we sure do have great days.

I would lie if I was to say that journalizing is easy. It definitely was not. However, I feel incredibly strong and proud knowing that I was able to do this and come out of the cocoon feeling like such a different person. A stronger, more independent, reconstructed individual with a whole lot more power to change the outcome of my life by having the tools to change myself, instead of trying to change others. What a relief!

—Hilda—

Sometime ago I made a list of the boundaries I wanted in my relationship with Mike. It has made it infinitely easier to deal with him in a civil manner and I feel healthier. He may never be aware of what the boundaries are . . . but as long as I know and maintain them, I am okay with where our relationship is at. I feel that now that I know what my boundaries are in this relationship, I need to work on my most important relationship, that with myself.

I feel that my most important work was in the second part of my matrix. I looked at how I wanted to define myself through the losses and then the gains, but, I don't feel that all negative or positive is how I wanted to define myself and my boundaries. I think that the most important gain was a redefining of my values and as I wrote and re-read the list I know this is what I needed to do to help guide me the rest of my life.

My Value System:

1. I express feelings openly and honestly with safe people.
2. I acknowledge reality.
3. I trust myself and my feelings.
4. I don't accept responsibility for the feelings of others.
5. I have choices.

6. I do not fear other's feelings.
7. I respect myself.
8. I am open and honest in relationships.
9. I am an equal in relationships.
10. I accept myself.
11. I accept others as they are.
12. I am humble.
13. I protect myself.
14. I don't accept responsibility for other's actions.
15. I take care of my needs.
16. I express anger appropriately in safe ways.
17. I connect with those I love.
18. I acknowledge my accomplishments.
19. I accept and love myself.
20. I maintain my boundaries.
21. I practice healthy sexuality.
22. I am honest.
23. I am responsible for myself.
24. I allow others to handle their own relationships.
25. I acknowledge my limits and ask for help.
26. I am aware of my needs and feelings.
27. I protect myself and my children from abusive behavior.
28. I am responsible for my behavior.
29. I minimize contact with toxic people.
30. I make my wants known.
31. I acknowledge my God.
32. I acknowledge my POWER.

—John—

Codependence is a disease that almost destroyed my soul. It invaded every part of my being—my professional life, my leisure time, my home life, my familial relationships and ultimately my relationship with my God.

My father died in the summer of 2000 and so began my unexpected, turbulent, and ultimately life-giving inner journey. With one phone call, my life was forever changed. I was suddenly very aware that I was living in a world of intense fear, depression, self-doubt, and that I was rapidly plummeting downward. I had to do something and do it fast.

I decided to call a highly-recommended counselor in town and luckily she was able to see me. She was warm, insightful and very caring. At the same time, she was direct, strong in her convictions and very clear about the therapeutic process. Together, we began looking at my relationships with my mother, father, friends, and religious community. She helped me delve into experiences that I had long buried and that had caused me so much despair, isolation, and fear. Fear was the dominating factor in my life at that point—fear of sickness, death, people, events and life in general. Simply put, I was afraid to die and even more afraid to live.

As the months passed I began doing inner child work. Initially, I remember hearing a voice within me saying, "no more, no more pain." Speaking with my counselor, she told me about the inner child and introduced me to the world of "left-hand" writing as a means of accessing the unconscious through the inner child. It gave me access to a world within that I never knew existed. As Carl Jung put it,

"In every adult, there lurks a child-an eternal child, something that is always becoming and is never completed and calls for necessary care, attention and education. That is part of the human personality which wants to develop and be whole."

Clearly, my inner child was crying out for recognition, healing and wholeness. My inner child, as I discovered slowly, was alive, creative, hiding, demanding attention, playful and punishing. Carl Jung's words now made perfect sense to me and I had no choice but to forge deeper and deeper into my own Inner Self.

The months passed and one day my counselor told me she believed I was ready for yet another step in the process of healing. What could that be, I wondered? She told me she thought I was ready to join a journaling group that met once a week to share the journey of self-discovery and inner healing. Initially, I was reluctant to join for fear someone in the group would recognize me; I did not want anyone to know that I was in this process or that I was going through so much pain. In actuality, there was someone who joined the group and did know me but that ultimately made the experience richer.

The group work involved looking at experiences, many from childhood that hurt us deeply, assaulted our values system, forced us to respond unhealthily to life's challenges, and ultimately robbed us of our identity and self-worth. Each week we shared very personal and painful experiences and slowly but surely, we saw ourselves taking greater risks in expressing strong and often long-buried emotions with less fear.

Nothing happens by accident. Looking back, every person played a role in my growth and I played a significant role in theirs. We belonged together! I saw each person laugh, cry, express tremendous anger, and cry out in despair. I saw tremendous love and support offered and accepted. I saw incredible courage-the courage to take a hard look at oneself and attempt to change. The group labored to confront the hurts and pain of their past and find ways to respond differently in the future. It was hard work but worthwhile work and we all knew it. The group process was helping us to grow albeit painfully.

Taking a more in-depth look at the content of my own inner work, I began with my relationship to my mother. Later, I tackled my relationship to my father again looking at particular incidents that hurt me, how I reacted then, my feelings, how the behavior contradicted my value system, how my present behavior was influenced by those events and betrayed my present value system and the losses to my identity. I remember the fear I felt as I looked at those events and the liberation I experienced as I got free of them. That was and is a great deal of work. Nonetheless, it was life-changing for the group.

Anger was a major issue for me. I had little ability to voice anger properly. I simply buried it. Needless to say, in my therapeutic process it all came bubbling up with a vengeance. The group process allowed me to look at it without fear or embarrassment because we were all in the same boat together. In fact, unlike anywhere else, getting in touch and exhibiting anger was encouraged and supported. That was so different from my family of origin or my work where anger was denied, hidden or misplaced.

My inner child work was bringing up loads of anger and the group was a safe place to share. Without that group, I do not know how I would have survived such a torrent of anger. The group was my processing haven and I am deeply grateful for that and to all of them. The group kept me honest when they thought I was denying my anger or rationalizing it by letting those who hurt me off the hook. Likewise, the group provided me a place where I could laugh and realize that despite it all, the sun would still come up tomorrow and as Julian of Norwich would often say, "all would be well." My approach to life was becoming lighter and in large measure, I had my group to thank for it.

It was very hard for me to deal with the "truth" of my parents. Because they were good in so many ways, I could not conceive of "betraying" them by speaking of their faults and failings and in a public forum, no less. With the help of the group, I came to realize that even good people can make serious mistakes and do "not so good things." It didn't matter whether they intended to do them or not. They did them and their actions affected me. I needed to acknowledge that before I could recover. My group was helpful in pointing out when I was "covering up, apologizing for, or protecting" the unhealthy behavior my parents exhibited toward me. While I didn't always like it, it was what I needed. They kept me honest and helped me to heal faster than I might have had I not been in their number.

Religion played an important role in my life and still does. I spent many years as a Roman Catholic religious in a community devoted to the Christian education of young people. It was a noble vocation and one that satisfied me for many years. Ultimately, I chose to leave the community after twenty-six years. The group process coupled with talk therapy and spiritual direction helped me to arrive at a place where I could courageously move on. It wasn't easy but it was what I was called to do. Throughout the time I spent in the journaling group, the group continuously encouraged me to be true to my Self no matter what the cost. That encouragement helped me to change my life for the better.

Ironically, my vocation as a Roman Catholic religious also had a profound effect on two group members. When I arrived in the group, I never mentioned that I had anything to do with the Catholic Church. I was simply a "school administrator". The longer I sat in the group, the more aware I became that two women in the group were deeply wounded by "church men" and very angry about it. One had been divorced from an ex-priest and the other was shamed by a priest and her Irish-Catholic family when she divorced her abusive husband. Her extremely Catholic family made her feel like a sinner and an outcast. Eventually, I told the group that I was a Roman Catholic minister and in both cases, the women remarked to me privately that my presence in the journaling group, especially as a Catholic minister, had brought some healing to their relationship with the Church and especially with men in the Church. One of the women remarked to me that "your presence in the group especially as a Roman Catholic religious has shown me another face of my Church and God—a softer, kinder, more loving God." Indeed, nothing happens by accident!

I must admit these women did cause me to think about why I remain in a religion that sometimes takes positions that seem out of touch with the modern world, can be dismissive of women, and are sometimes shamefully lacking in compassion for the marginalized and those who just can't live what the Church teaches. Since I left the journaling group, many women and men have challenged me similarly and I consider that a good thing. Given these authentic challenges, why do I stay a member of an organized religion, in my case the Roman Catholic Church, and how has my continued membership in the Church helped me to grow spiritually?

First, the Church continues to be filled with some truly "modern-day Saints", men women who inspire me to stay close to Jesus Christ and continue to proclaim, mostly by example, Jesus' Good News. Clearly, the world needs that more than ever. Second, I need support in seeking God. I need a community of faith and with all its imperfections and faults, I still find it in the Church. Like my family of origin, I may not like everything about the Roman Catholic Church, but it's still mine and I still love it. Third, much of my recovery has been based on the twelve steps. The concept of a Higher Power (which I conceive as God) continues to be helpful to my recovery process and the Church supports me in that process. Fourth, the lives of the Saints throughout history continue to show me viable ways of "seeking God in a broken world." Finally, the celebration of the Eucharist continues to nourish me and gives me strength for the journey.

The journaling group process had a profound effect on me. It clarified my need for support and validated the pain I was hiding deep within. It helped me confront my rage and express it in a safe, loving environment. It provided a disciplined, systematic way to deal with my inner child and to find out what was needed to bring myself to wholeness. It allowed me to experience the struggles of others and realize that I was not the only one feeling this way. It taught me patience with My Self when tempted to say, "Oh, just get over it." The group taught me how foolish and damaging such a statement can be for self and others!

My counselor played a significant role in our journaling group. She kept us focused, faithful to the process and just plain honest with ourselves and one another. She was perceptive, insightful and compassionate. Make no mistake about it; she could also be brutally honest when necessary and I always appreciated that quality in her. Without her support, we could not have journeyed to the inner places where we needed to go. I will be forever grateful that she came my way.

Today, I am far more confident in my abilities as a professional and an adult person. I am less intent upon getting the approval of others and more intent on listening first to my own inner truth. If my inner truth and doing what others want coincides, that's great! If not, I am less inclined to simply please the other and hurt My Self. Believe me, I have a long way to go in this regard but I can safely say I have come a long way thanks to my journaling group. I know my self-esteem has improved dramatically. I went from a frightened little boy in a man's body to a more confident man secure in his identity and clearer on both his gifts and his limitations. The journaling group provided the bridge necessary to go from one to the other.

I continue to pursue therapy as a means to personal and professional growth. Life continues to have its challenges and its blessings. Two years ago, I lost my only nephew at nineteen years of age. This tossed me into a world of grief, pain, and the grueling process of letting go. I continue in that process today. I have certainly had my challenges at work and in relationships but I am better able to negotiate them because of the lessons learned in my journaling group. I have lots of love in my life and I am much better able to just have fun. I enjoy life more.

Years ago, I used to think that going to therapy would result in an eventual cure. The words of Carl Rodgers bring me encouragement as a "cure" never came. Rodgers reminds me that "the good life is a process, not a state of being. It is a direction and not a destination." Involvement in my journaling group set me in a direction and I realize that is the best one can hope for and probably all one needs-a journey of ups and downs leading one closer and closer to self, others, God. Confident that "nothing happens by accident", I continue my life's journey with gratitude for the past and confidence in the future.

—Mickael—

I came to this country, the United States of America at the age of 31 with a pregnant wife and my dearest eldest daughter, full of emotion and plans for the future, ready to make it in the U.S.A. One problem though: I had few clues of who I was. Of course, I thought I knew.

This country represented many years of dreaming. I was born in a very large family, with brothers and sisters as well as many cousins, uncles and extended family. It was easy to be overlooked and to be able to do what I wanted, in some cases not to my best advantage.

Being from a large family it was not easy for all of us all the time. But I had a very good childhood. My father, a professional, made a good living but moved us to a larger city. He commuted once a week from another city where he worked. He spent weekends with us. My mother would run things around the house until my father came on the weekend. We were expected to behave and not give my mother any problems. In the summers, we went back to the city where my father worked. That was great; the mountains, the river, the camping and the stars of my mother's town got into me and became part of me. But in winter, I missed my father. I longed for attention and direction. I know now how much I missed my father while he was away. I drifted in and out trying to find who I was and what I wanted in life. Overall though, we did not go without any physical needs, though nurturing came a bit scarce; there were many siblings to take care of. Nature, sports and studying to our highest potential was expected, there was not much tolerance for rudeness or impoliteness. Religious education was part of our everyday life. With so many brothers and sisters, I still felt lonely, and at times isolated.

It was not until I came to this country and after my first divorce from my late high-school sweetheart and already into my second marriage, that I realized that I was an alcoholic. It was not obvious because I had not had any arrest or DWI or violent behavior. Some would say that I had never been drunk.

My addiction was more subtle, much more cunning and baffling to me. I drank to be able to disinhibit myself, to lie to myself. A couple of beers or a scotch could be enough to engage me in bad behavior. My religious upbringing made me regret very fast every time that I lied or was untruthful. When it happened, I rationalized it and told myself that it had been a mistake to do this or that . . . that it had only happened a couple of times . . . that I knew I would not do it again. Bottom line, I could not make the connection between being a bit "high" and my bad behavior. But that small amount of alcohol was enough to cause me to do things I did not want to do . . . and I could not help it. Isn't it that the definition of addiction?

Things were not easy for my first wife either. By the time we got married, she was no longer in love with me. I wanted children, she didn't. She wanted solitude, I was gregarious. I needed a relationship, she did not need one. She got depressed and left for a few months. She came back and we got divorced. I was angry and terrified and resolute about taking care of my girls. I changed cities and became a single parent, my second daughter still in diapers. I had several relationships before my second marriage.

So in my second marriage, which lasted a bit more than nine years, problems started to flourish from the very beginning. I buried myself in a ton of work and promised myself to be honest in this relationship. My relationship with my second wife had good and bad moments, but in order to save the marriage I accepted something that I will regret the rest of my life. I sent my two daughters from my previous marriage to live with their mother. I had been a single parent since my first divorce. I was not attentive to their emotional needs . . . I will talk about this at a different time.

But problems continued and I had no idea why. I was a good provider; I had accepted a child from my second wife and treated him as my own. I was loving towards all my children and I had a third daughter in my second marriage, whom I adore. So therapy started: I have to say that we probably went to ten therapists over the course of different cities where we lived and in the nine years of our marriage. Every time that I started to make some progress, my wife or I would derail the process, arguing that the therapist was siding with one of us. In trying to save the marriage I would go along with the changes. This is how we met my dear therapist; my ex-wife introduced me to her. The therapist had a condition not to drink while we were undergoing therapy. That was easy for me; alcohol was not my problem . . .

So my dear therapist started very slowly with individual therapy and then suggested that I enter group therapy. She thought that I needed to work on the bad experience of my first marriage. My first wife, during her depression had left me with two daughters. My upbringing had a lot to do with how I got to be who I was. I had to tell the therapy group how badly my first wife had treated me. That was part of the process; as I started to see my reaction at that mistreatment I started to see my self destructive behavior. During my first marriage, I became a workaholic. I needed her to function . . . and deceit took place. I violated my values and that took a toll on me, a downward spiral that could only be broken by accepting that I had a problem. But that took some time to accept.

What I didn't realize, was that working on my first marriage was the tip of the iceberg. As I continued with therapy, I had the opportunity to see how a dominating father and a submissive mother created patterns that I learned. At times, I could endure anything for the sake of my present marriage and at other times I would get on my high horse (yelling and screaming) if things didn't go my way. Through my therapy, I found fault with how my parents raised us. Later, I realized with profound understanding, what good people they were and that they did their best. They loved us in a way that only good parents can. I found my mother's strength in her quietness and smiling calmness. I saw her inner strength. I saw and understood my father's upbringing and how loving he was to all of us. My mother was able to love without any resentment and my father was a loving man to his wife, like no other man I know. My parents' relationship deserves a complete story that I will avoid for right now. This is a story of love, strength, integrity, and faith.

My dear therapist then had me work on the current marriage at the time, my second wife. But the process to get to a better state of mind was the same as before and very long. First feel what had happened; scream, punch a pillow, and kick that boxing mannequin, and write, write, write . . . then again to realize my reaction to the real abuse, because it was real emotional abuse that I felt. That abuse damaged me and I later learned that my reaction had violated my values. And my reaction took another route, manipulation of my wife, through threats, divorce and finally depression. This was a vicious cycle between both of us. Months at a time without a loving relationship proved too much for me. I became very depressed; the contrast of not feeling loved and not seeing a way out proved too much for me. I became a puppet to my wife. I lost all power.

Therapy and the great support system of men that had gone through similar situations sustained me. By the Grace of God, early breakfast with good friends, meetings, and working on my co-dependency through therapy pulled me through.

I remember one day that I had suicidal thoughts. Was I trying to manipulate her into having her love me? Probably, but the suicidal thoughts were real. The pain that day was so great that I phoned my best friend at the time and told him about my situation. He asked me to come to his apartment and on his knees prayed to God in front of me, with tears in his eyes; he asked God to take care of me and to remove those feelings from me.

I remember that a big burden, a dark cloud on top of me had been lifted. I was almost laughing. And in a few days my depression went away gradually. Then another epiphany . . . I was freer and freer from manipulation . . . Through all of this I stayed sober and more importantly, I was truthful. Then I started to really change and became more honest and less dependent on other people, especially my second wife. The rubber band of our relationship was stretched to the limit . . . I could not be manipulated like before. I took up golf, I administered food to the homeless, I read, and enjoyed male friendships like never before. I got closer to my parents and my daughters. I could start letting go with love. Then after 3 attempts back and forth at getting divorced we finally divorced. I left the house with very little, but I was free from becoming a bad person.

Through my second marriage, I kept my values where they mattered most. I could not have done it without the friends and meetings that supported me. Through the process I realized that the problem did not reside in others. It resided in me all along. It had to do with my ex-wives, my upbringing, missed opportunities and lack of direction but it had to do more with how I responded to the mistreatment and how I violated my values.

Once alone, after my divorce, I started to feel even better. Then after several relationships in the course of several years, I met my present wife. Yes, I am in my third marriage.

God gave me several gifts and put me through the trial of my life all at the same time; my second daughter came to live with me for almost two years before God claimed her. She was very sick with anorexia nervosa. After her death the pain was excruciating, greater that I can possibly explain and it was when my little one told me; "Dad, promise me that you won't die on me"; the little one was worried about me, but that is another story of grief in my life that I won't go into detail today. Previous patterns of behavior came back, but I did not drink. I knew that drinking would be a recipe for dishonesty.

Anything associated with my daughter's death took a different twist. My life was shattered to pieces. In the course of almost four years I lost two jobs, my mother passed away, had several relationships with women, but could not hold on to a relationship.

Life changed and brought good things to me. I met my present wife. My eldest daughter came to live with me, what a blessing! I got another job that I love. This job sent me close to where my father lived in the old continent. I saw him every month for over a year and a half and there after at least 3 times a year for several years. God brought me closer to my father and I got closer to him. I never doubted the love I felt for my mother but I had felt distant from my father even though I would talk to him every week since I left to the US. God allowed me to meet my father in another way and I was able to talk to him man to man. I know today how much he loved me and how much I love him. I started to feel my parent's protection from above. Certainly I had had that feeling from my mother all along.

Today I have found peace, I feel no hate. Though, once in a while, if I feel as if I am getting out of whack, I go to my tool box and recite to myself: is it really important enough to get upset? When I point a finger at someone, am I not pointing three fingers at me? Is it really about me? What is it about the serenity prayer I do not get at this time? Live and let live, exercise, talk about it, write, go to church, go to a meeting, be with my friends, my wife. Am I hungry, angry, lonely or tired? Then eat, talk about it, meet a friend or rest. Certainly what I love the best is being with my wonderful wife. I have never felt better around a woman.

I pray and look at my life and there are always things to ask for forgiveness to God and to another human being. So I go through my 12 steps and if I lie to myself, I eventually know.

I am married to the most beautiful person I have ever known. I live accepting of life with scars in my soul, but sober, and with willingness to do well and maximize goodness around me. That is my motto Maximize Goodness everywhere I am.

Dedicated to my therapist

Example Of A
Closure Letter:

John,

It is time for me to say good-bye. Knowing you has been the greatest joy to begin and the deepest hell toward the end. And now that all has been said and done, I am grateful for the experience.

It was inspiring, moving, frightening, and disconcerting that time with you.

I see my part in this drama we played out and the lessons learned were mine. So it is with gratitude that I can now say farewell . . . to the anger, resentment, pain, that was still a bond between us. I feel no need to be linked to you in any way.

So this is a joyful farewell. In knowing you and the experiences we shared, I am now able to make new choices, explore new horizons, able to live an exceptional life free of expectations and full of expectancy . . . free of limits. For this I thank you. I wish you well.

Dear Derrick:

I am writing this letter to you so that you may have a glimpse of what my life has become without you.

Over the 32 years of our time together, I discovered the real you. Unfortunately, a very selfish, work-driven, money-making machine. This reality turned our lives into chaos. Your lack of caring, support, intimacy, honesty, faithfulness and parenting pushed me into seeking guidance through my therapy, support groups, journaling and 12-step recovery work. I learned to: stand on my own as a single woman; parent and to literally protect, defend, support and raise our children. How sad it is that you chose the dark path of negativity, to continue not seeking guidance, to repeat the behaviors of your father and ultimately destroy our family. The good news is: I am a new person! I am stronger now and happier than I can ever remember! You didn't break me! I have become a loving, trusting, self-respecting, confident and secure woman. And, I'm so happy to say that I've moved forward with my life and am so excited about all the new possibilities on my own.

Kristine

Looking Back

In January 2003, he stood in front of a mirror in an old house in Chester, PA. He was up before his roommate and well before the rest of the inmates. He peeled back his eyelids and forced himself to look at the man looking back at him. There was a shadow and a demon blocking the view of the person on the inside. The outside looked nothing like the creature in the shadow on the inside. Of the twelve residents, one was black, one was gay, two were old, two were very young. One was Hispanic and two were Jews. One was tattooed from head to toe. Each one was placed with him by God to work with him to find a way through. All of them shared a bond and all of them shared a disease, a progressive, terminal disease, if not treated and taken seriously. All of them were angry and resentful.

They had all come from different locations at different ages but all had reached the same place at this particular time. Looking back, they said it wasn't going to be easy. Looking back, they said if you want what we have, you have to be willing to go to any length to get it. Looking back, all of them relapsed, half of them continued on, one died, two lost professional licenses, two divorced, and two went to prison. Looking back, they all believed they were victims and they all believed they were the center of the universe. Looking back, they said there was a program of recovery.

Twelve steps led the way to a lifetime of peace and serenity. There were those less fortunate who failed but only did so because they were incapable of telling the truth.

Looking back, they said the truth will set you free. Looking back, they said this recovery would be hard work. Many looked for a softer, gentler way, but that did not work. The result would be nil unless they let go absolutely. Looking back, they said there were promises.

The fear of people and economic insecurity would leave, they promised we would lose interest in selfish things and gain interest in our fellows. We would intuitively know how to handle situations which used to baffle us. They promised we would realize that God was doing for us what we could not do for ourselves. Looking back, these don't look extravagant. They are being fulfilled among us, sometimes quickly, sometimes slowly. They will always materialize if we are willing to work for them. Looking back, there was a world of pain, a path of destruction. Looking back, there were her tears, their disappointment. Looking back, there were many amends, many not fulfilled because to do so would hurt others. Looking back, there was a loving counselor who gave away what she had in order to get it back. She said to find the God of your understanding and find faith in Him. She said to take what you want and leave the rest. Looking back, she said to find a sponsor, in fact, she had the right one already picked out for me and said it was a God thing. Looking back, she said keep coming back it works if you work it and you are worth it. Looking back, she said let go and let God. Looking back, she said she had a group to work with to work through resentment and anger. Looking back, she said to forgive them. She said, they didn't have the tools, they did the best they could. Looking back, she filled a tool box for all to use free of charge anytime one is needed. They get sharper each time they are used and shared. Looking back, she said do ninety meetings in ninety days, and over seven years there were fourteen hundred. There were several groups, many new friends, three journals, sponsors, referrals, and many, many days of peace and serenity. Looking back, she said it is never over, take it one day at a time. She said my door is open; you have a safe place when you need it. Looking back, hey, look who is looking back! It is me looking back at me in the mirror. The outside looks a lot like the inside. Keep coming back, it works when you work it and it is worth it. Looking back, God has blessed me in so many ways. I have an attitude of gratitude and I have so many to thank and so much to give away in order to receive.

God bless you and thank you for saving my life.